Intermediate Pole Dancing

For Fitness and Fun

By

Danni Peck

Intermediate Pole Dancing: For Fitness and Fun

Copyright © 2017

ISBN-10: 1521190763

ISBN-13: 978-1521190760

Warning and Disclaimer

Every effort has been made to make this book as accurate as possible. However, no warranty or fitness is implied. The information provided is on an "as-is" basis. The author and the publisher shall have no liability or responsibility to any person or entity with respect to any loss or damages that arise from the information in this book.

Publisher contact

Skinny Bottle Publishing

books@skinnybottle.com

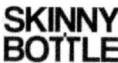

Introduction to Intermediate Pole Dancing

You've probably gotten familiar with your pole at this point and this is great! However, do you feel like taking it further? That's where this book comes in. This book will tell you all about some of the amazing intermediate pole moves that you can learn and perfect.

Starting with pole dancing is usually a huge first step, and you have taken that. You know how to do basic spins, basic moves, and the like. But what about some of the other moves you see? What about those pretty moves you see in various pole videos online that make you go, "Hey, I really want to do that!" Well, you can. This book will take you through what you need to know about the intermediate moves.

Now, these moves will take a bit longer to learn. It's not because they're super complex, but they have a different feel. You'll have to overcome some basic fears you might have of the pole and we'll go over those fears later. It's completely justified, and you might initially not want to try these intermediate moves simply because of how scary they might be. But don't despair, nor should you worry. Instead, read this book, learn about the techniques, and from there, start to pole dance for success and learn some of the killer intermediate moves.

This is your next step, and I do believe in you. You've got this! Make sure that you do take the time to learn more; to learn all that you need so that you can pole for success. You'll definitely feel amazing by the time you finish this book and learn the moves outlined in here.

All About the Invert

The first thing that you should learn when it comes to intermediate techniques is the invert. This is going upside down and it's the key part of many people's ascensions into learning more difficult moves. However, it's important to note that this move is not easy.

This move might be one of the hardest moves that you'll start out with, because not only does it require a ton of actual physical strength, but you need to have mental strength as well. You might feel fear the moment you start to see the pole and the idea of hanging upside down might utterly terrify you. However, that's totally normal, and we'll go into that fear in more detail later on.

Nothing to Fear but Fear Itself

When you look at girls going upside down, the first thing you'll probably think is how utterly easy it is. Well, that's not the case. An invert takes a lot of strength for one, but it also takes a bit of guts and an ability to confront and face your fears.

For many, the idea of hanging upside down might seem easy initially, but it's often kind of scary the moment you try to do it. That's because you almost feel like you might fall, and often, that fear of falling might be the difference between hanging upside down successfully ... or not. However, there really isn't a reason to worry all that much, for you can train yourself to overcome this fear.

The best way to overcome this fear is to just keep doing the trick. With inverts, you might do this about fifty times before you finally get it, and you might feel a bit scared initially. However, don't worry. Just keep doing this again and again. You'll see the difference in no time. Often, if you practice this at least 5-

10 times each session and then go back to your other exercises, you'll feel much better.

With inverts, it's good to also work on picking your legs up. You might be able to get them up, but you might struggle with that final part of the invert. If you need to, try to work on that, preparing your abs for the action at hand. Remember, this takes a lot of ab strength, so you should make sure your body is conditioned for this type of activity before you begin.

If you fear you're going to hurt yourself, put some cushions over the bottom area of your pole. That way, should you actually fall, you won't hurt yourself. If you're doing this on hardwood floors, it's highly recommended that you have something cushioning around the pole in case of these accidents.

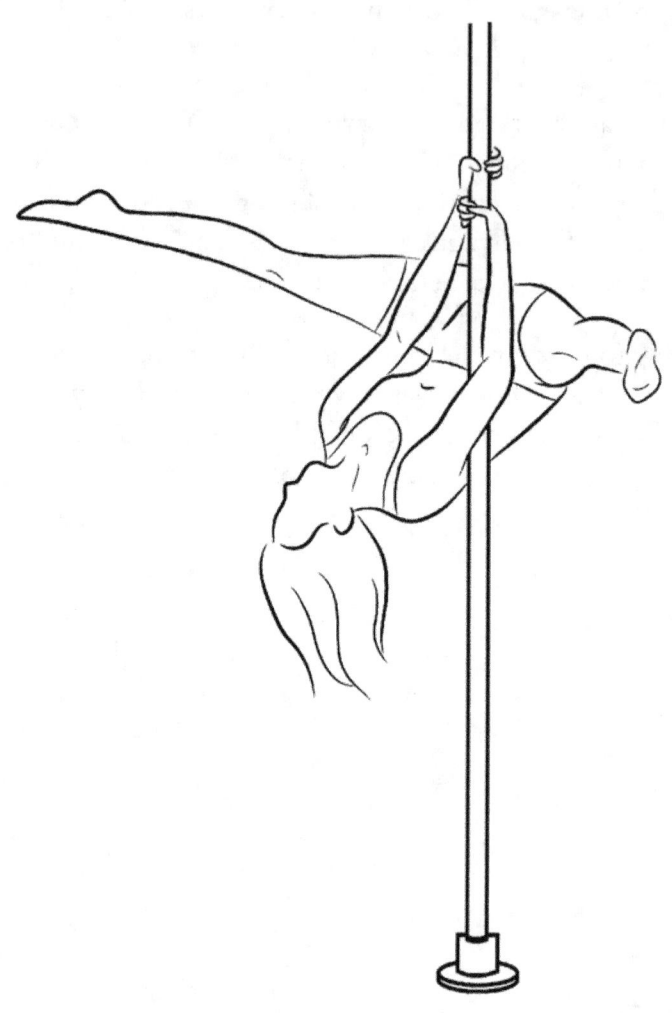

Abs are an Essential

When it comes to inverts, you need ab strength. Think about it. How are you going to kick your legs up and hold them there if you have no ab strength? It's important that you start building your abs, whether it be during your practice sessions, or at another time.

You should be targeting your lower abdominals. You might have some killer upper abs, but if your lower abs are weak, you won't be able to pick your feet up. It's as simple as that. To work on this, leg drops, partial leg drops, leg lifts, and planks help a lot. You should work on all your sets of abs period, but if you're looking to add a little extra to your ab workout, consider those before you attempt inverts.

How to Do an Invert

Now that you have a good grasp on what you're going to do next, it's time to work on the invert. You should ideally do this by sweeping the outside leg up and not trying to kick or do a running start. You should make sure that the weight goes from the back foot to the foot in front, and that the outside leg is almost swept up when you go. You would be working to do a pivot up, twisting your arms to pivot yourself up.

When you do sweep the leg up, this is where the ab strength comes in. You should make sure that the muscles are all working together in a very long line, almost like a plank, going from upright to inverted. You should try to pull down on the pole when you use your arms, almost pulling it to the crotch. You shouldn't be thinking about getting the legs to the pole, but instead, mastering how to get your crotch to the pole. Yes, this sounds crazy, but that is exactly how you should do it.

The movement should stop when the hips are at the pole, and when they are there, you should have them completely there. By this point, your weight should be almost vertical, and you should almost have the balance going upside down without even wrapping your legs. It should be easy for you if you have your hips all the way up. Once you're up in the air, sweep the leg over to the front of the pole to lock in.

If you tend to hook the ankle and then pull the crotch to the pole, you should break this habit by picking a spot about five feet above you and get the ankle to that place. If needed, tightly tie a scarf to that point and then keep everything close to the pole until your hips are almost overhead. You might feel weightless because you're pulling down while you're pulling up. If you straighten your arms before that, you're typically kicking up and not moving your butt up the pole. Make sure that you work on trying to get your crotch up to the pole. That's the priority.

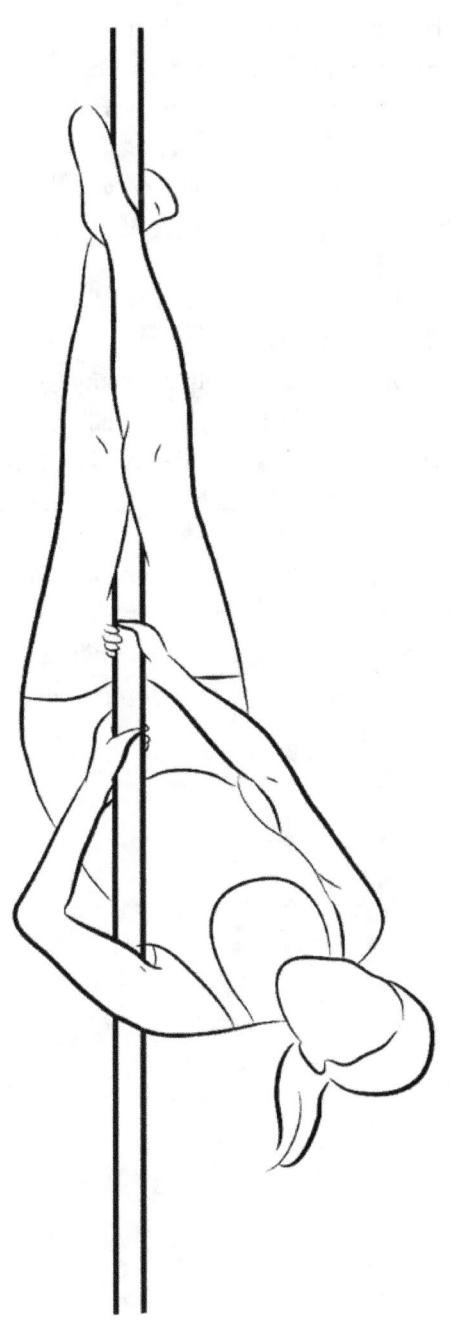

If you start to form the habit of moving behind the pole, it could mean trouble when you're trying to get your legs up and your hips straight on the pole. If you are away from where the pole is, or even arching yourself backward, you can't bend your body and hold yourself in the position. It makes it a lot harder, because your hips will move away from the pole and you'll only get your ankle on there. You should make sure that you're aware of this mistake in form.

Really, the key action here is to get your crotch to the pole. You should be close. You should be using that force to get yourself up there but if you're struggling with this, try to add in a bit of ab work to help fully engage your body. You'll be surprised at just what kind of a difference it will make on your body. If you are struggling with this, do try again and again. Remember, if you can't get your legs up, look at your position, for it could make all the difference.

This chapter went over how to perform one of the most amazing and probably scariest moves for you to begin with when you're pole dancing. Inverts are a key action to learn since many various parts of pole dancing involve this. Learn it, master it, and you'll soon see the difference as you proceed.

Intermediate Spins to Learn

There are other spins that you can learn. These ones are simple and yet very effective. If you've mastered the basics and want something slightly more complicated, then you've come to the right chapter. This chapter will go over just some of the best intermediate spins to learn when you're pole dancing.

Reverse Stag

Remember the stag spin from the beginner book? Well, there is a reverse to it. It's imperative that you know how to do the normal stag before you try the reverse, since it can be a bit more complicated. You'll have to rely far more on arm strength, too, to hold yourself up.

Essentially, it's a stag spin where you're going in a backward rotation versus a forward one. Your leg won't be hooked around the pole like a normal stag spin, but instead, your thigh will be against it. You'll have your arms holding yourself up and when ready, you can move your legs into that position, and then hold it there. It's a bit of a weird sort of feeling, mostly because it doesn't feel normal. Often, the biggest challenge is getting used to how this move feels before you do it, for it can feel slightly off.

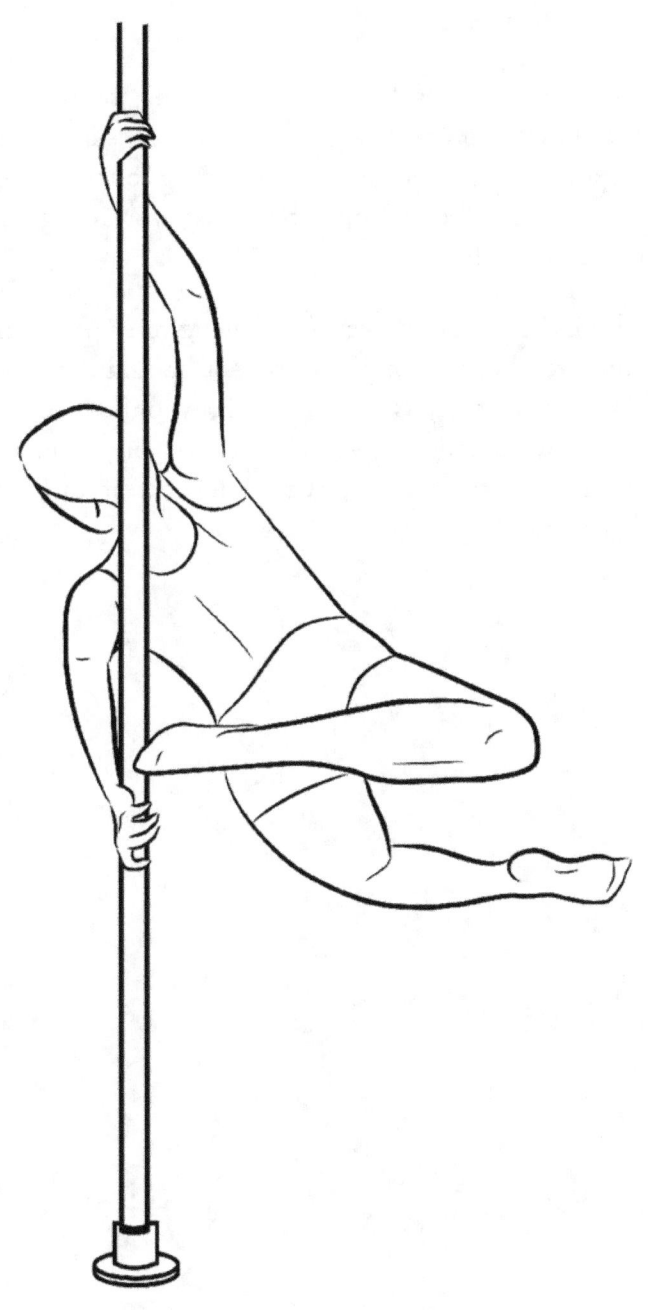

Chopper Spin

If you're a fan of hanging upside down and spinning, this is a great spin to learn. You also should work on pointing your toes. This is a common error many who start to pole dance forget about, but pointing your toes makes a difference in how pretty a move looks. You should first work on getting yourself up before you start to do this.

You should walk around the pole while having your inner arm holding it — similar to how you begin with an invert. You should then take your outside arm and hold it to the pole, use your abs to lift your body up just like how you would with an invert, and once you're inverted, you should extend your legs out and let your body go around the pole. This is great for your abdominals as well, as it is a big challenge.

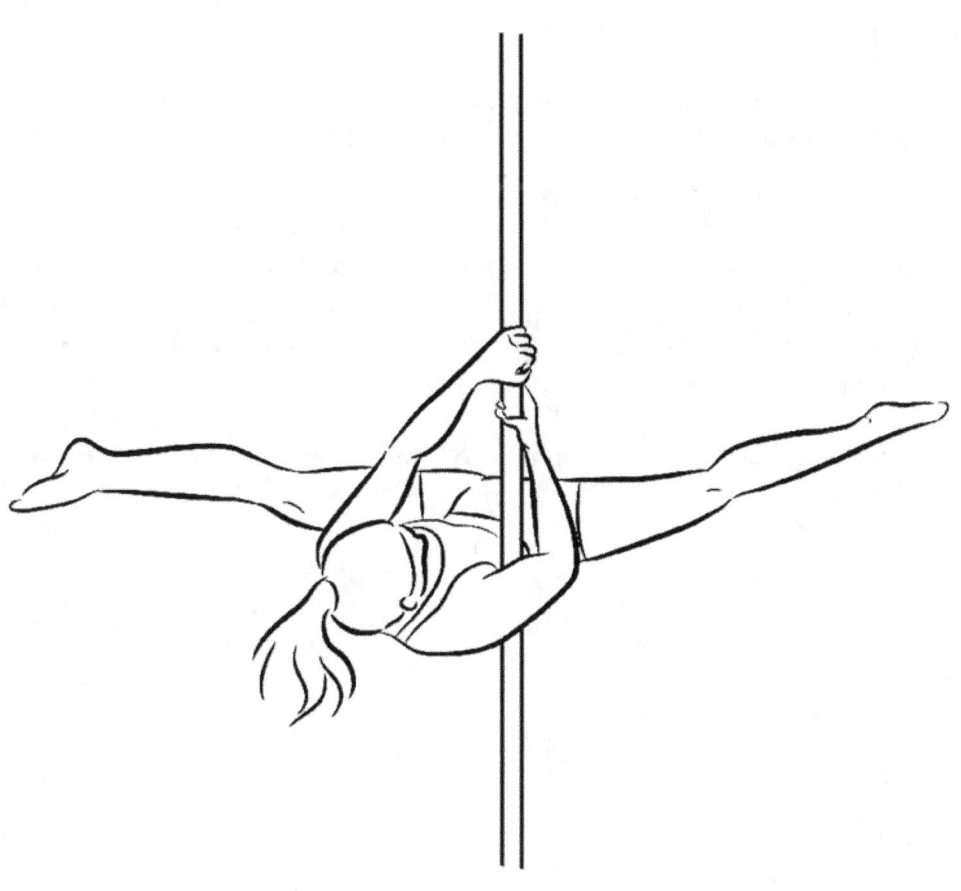

Straddled Carousel Spin

This is a great spin to learn if you want to create a pretty move with your legs still against the pole. You start this one by walking around the pole and having the inner arm gripping the pole. You should then take the arm outside and bring it up to a split grip, which is essentially holding your hands about a foot or two apart. You should then lift your legs up and hold them forward into a V shape. Your hands will be the primary supporter of your weight. You'll then point your toes to give this spin an added touch. This is great for arm strength as well.

Note that a split grip can be hard on your wrists, so approach this move carefully.

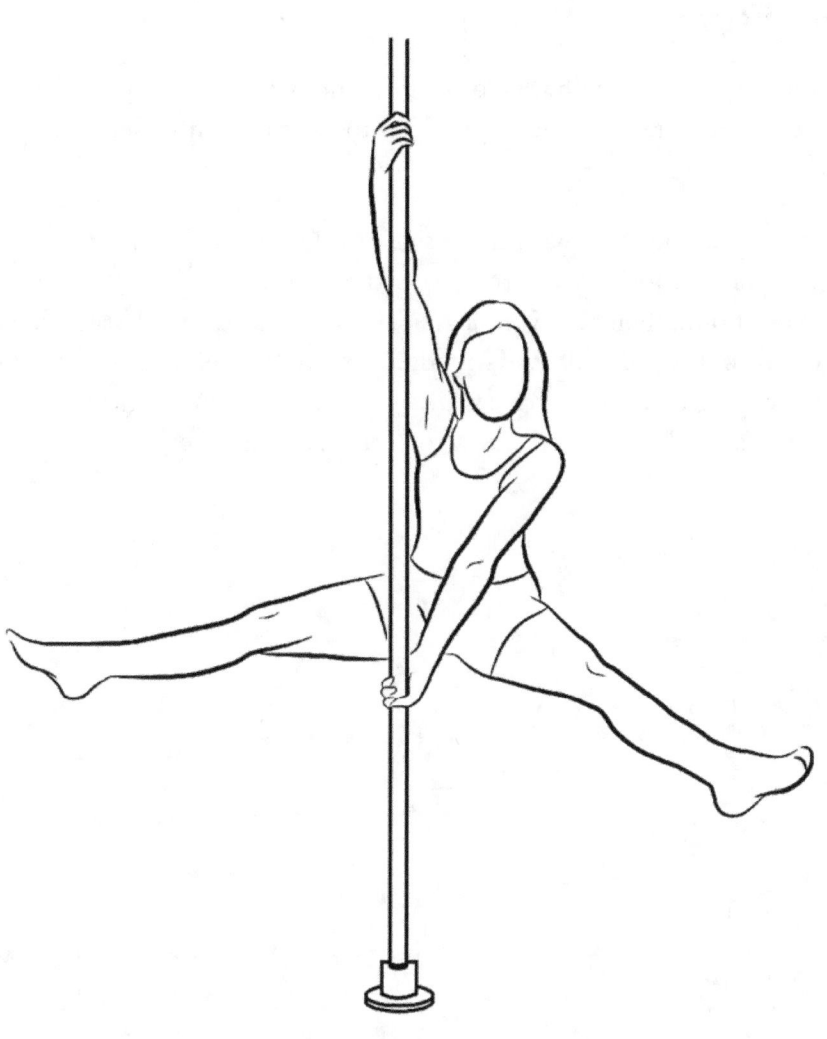

Fang Carousel Spin

This is another carousel spin that looks great and has a bit of extra challenge to it. You should notice with these spins that focus is certainly on arm grip and strength.

To start, you should walk with the inside arm holding the pole. You should then have your opposite arm brought to the pole in the split grip, just like before. You should then hold your legs up; however, instead of letting them go to either side of the pole (like the straddle), you should bend them behind you at the knee area. You should have your toes pointed. Your weight will still be against your arms, but it's a great way to create a better outer spin.

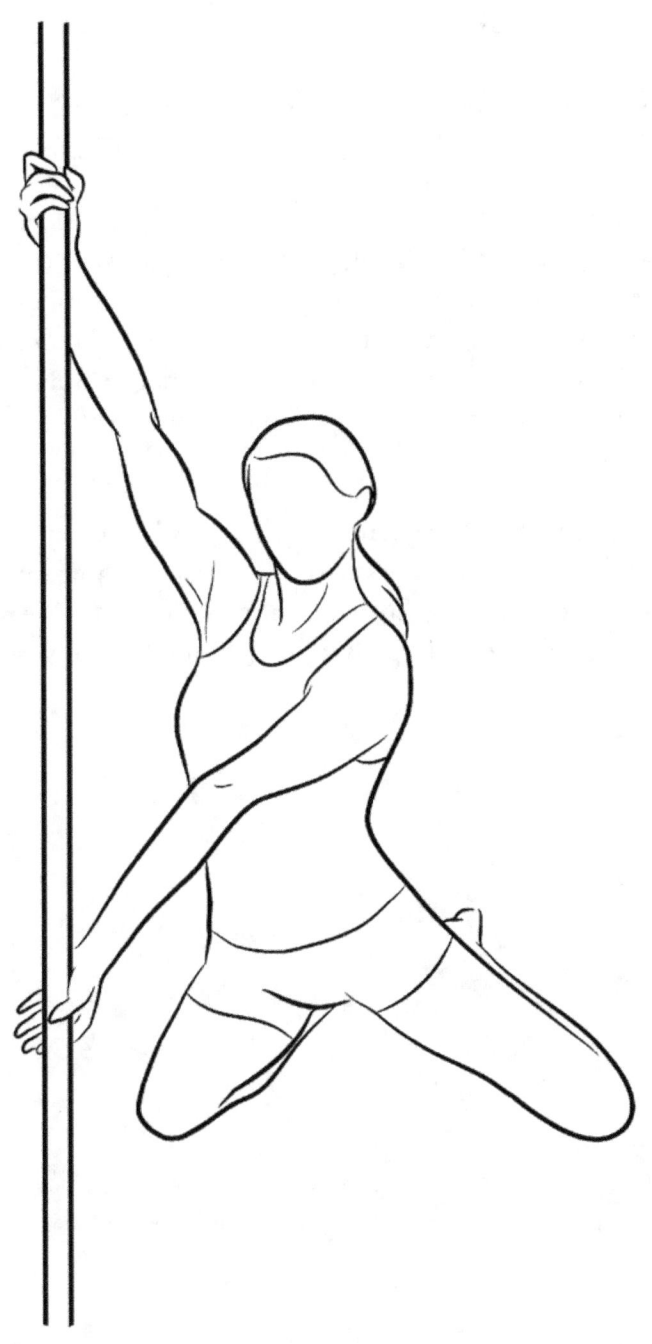

Back Spiral Spin

This is a spin that can look a bit awkward at first. However, once you get the hang of it, and your arm placements correct, it can look great.

To start this, you should walk around the pole with the inner arm gripping it. Now, instead of normally moving your outer leg forward or around, you will move your legs into the stag position. This is a bit weird at first, and you might feel silly, but practice at least lifting your feet off the ground and trying this. You should then have your outer arm grip the pole behind you, keeping the shoulders against the pole. You should point your toes while you do this and then arch your back.

Essentially, this is one of the harder ones, simply because getting your feet up like that and making it look aesthetically pleasing can be quite complicated. It's best that if you are struggling with this spin, to master the reverse stag spin before moving on. The back spiral spin builds up the reverse stag.

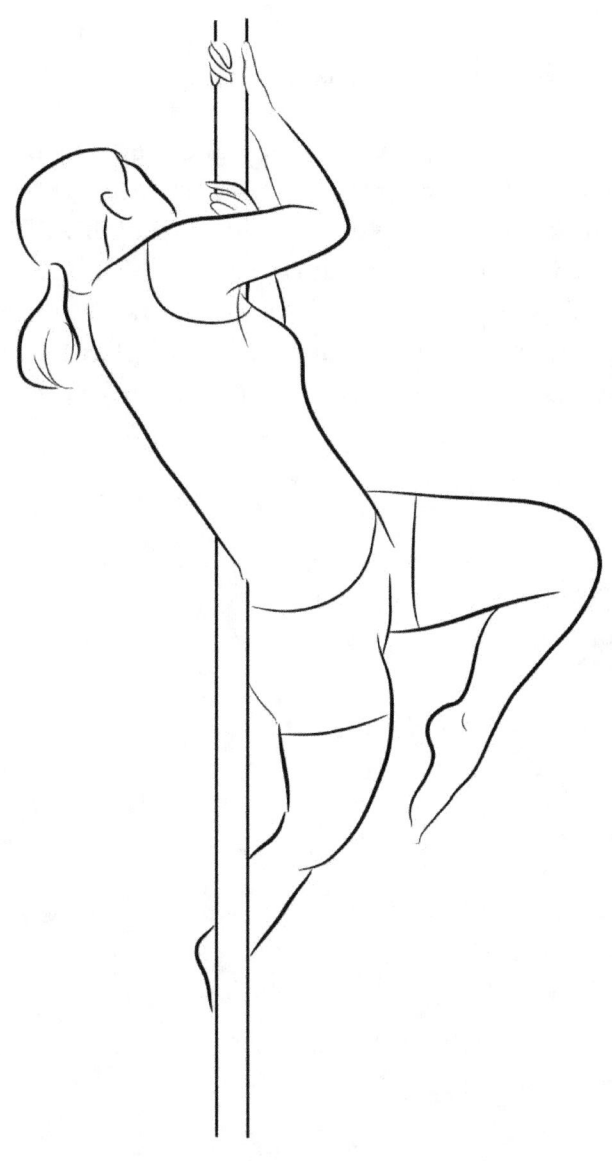

Side Spiral Spin

This is another fun spin, and you probably have seen this before. It's a great one to learn because other more complicated spins are built on it.

To start learning this, you should walk around the pole with your inside arm gripping the pole. You should then have your outside arm go to the pole as well, having it on the other side in a basic handspring grip. While holding this, you should then begin to make your body turn horizontally. You should tuck your legs in and from there, slowly loosen your grip as you move down the pole. The hand position, combined with bringing your feet up against there, can often be the biggest struggle, so make sure that you keep your abs engaged as you do this.

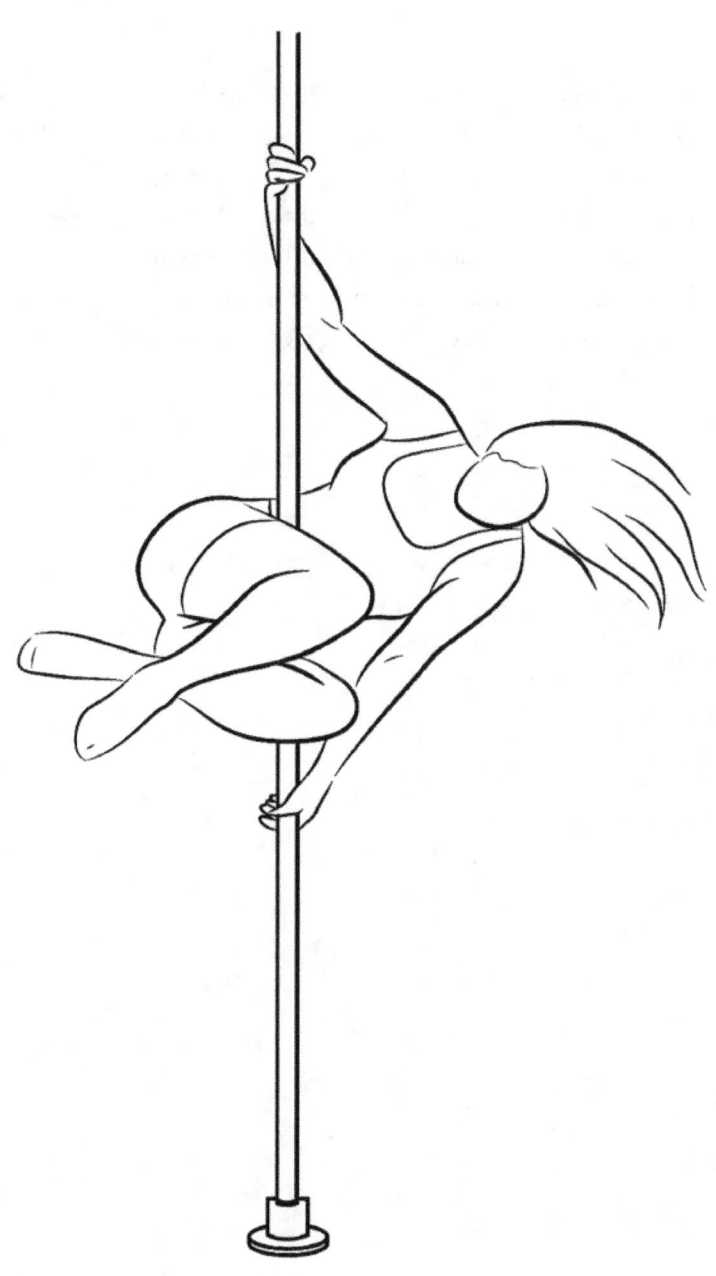

Low lift

This is a fun spin that takes some serious ab work. To do this, you should start on the floor with the knee closest to the pole in a kneeling position and your outer leg extended out into a side lunge. You should have your hands about six inches apart, gripping the akin to a baseball bat. You should then swing the leg that is outside around the pole and then hold your knee up off the floor. This will essentially put you in a variation of the side spiral spin. This is a much harder move and does require a very engaged core, so make sure you work on that.

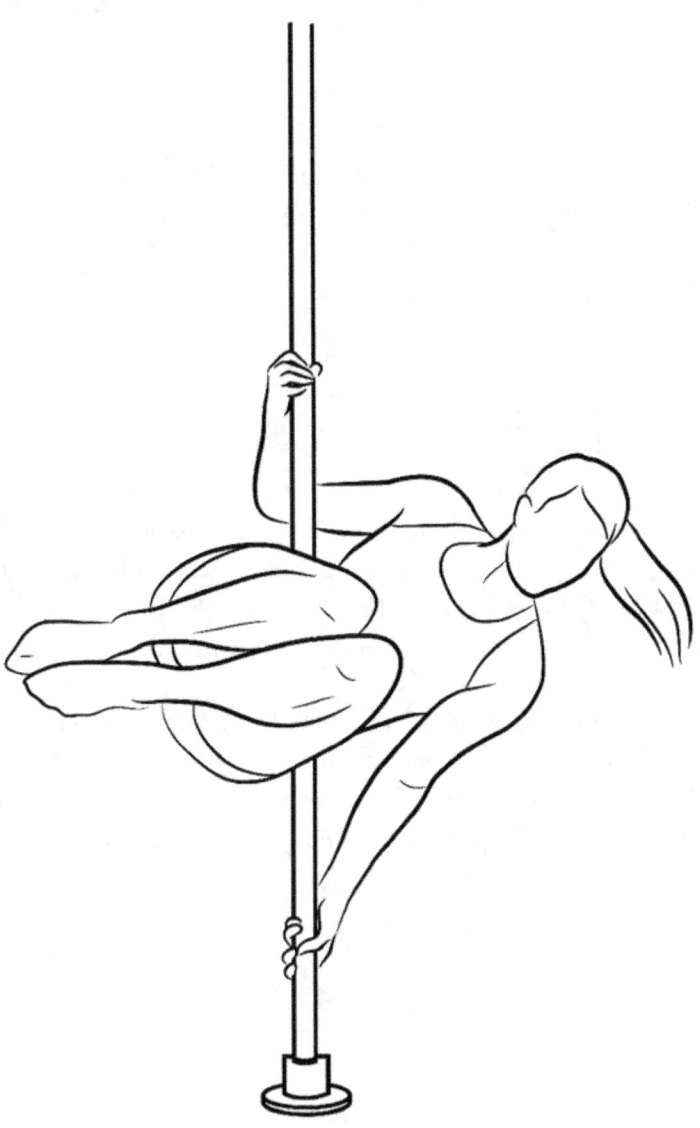

This chapter went over some of the harder spins that you can try. They might be complicated, but they are quite fun, so make sure you practice them a bit before you try them.

Intermediate Inversions to Practice

We went over how to do the basic inversion, now it's time to talk about some of the cool various inversion tricks you can do from here. Once you've gotten your body up from the ground to an inverted position, there's a lot that you can do. This chapter will go over what you can do in order to improve your pole dancing skills.

Extension of Basic

To do this, the first thing you should do is start with the basic inversion. From there, wrap your legs around the pole, crossing them at the ankles and gripping the pole hard between the legs. You can slowly loosen this grip to slide down. Make sure to tuck your head in though, since you can hurt your head and neck.

A word of caution with inverts is that when you do these, you'll feel the burn. You might even get a few bruises as well. If you weren't sore before, you might be at the end of attempting this move. It's important to not give up but build from that. You won't be hurting forever and conditioning the skin to holding your body up like that is integral to your success.

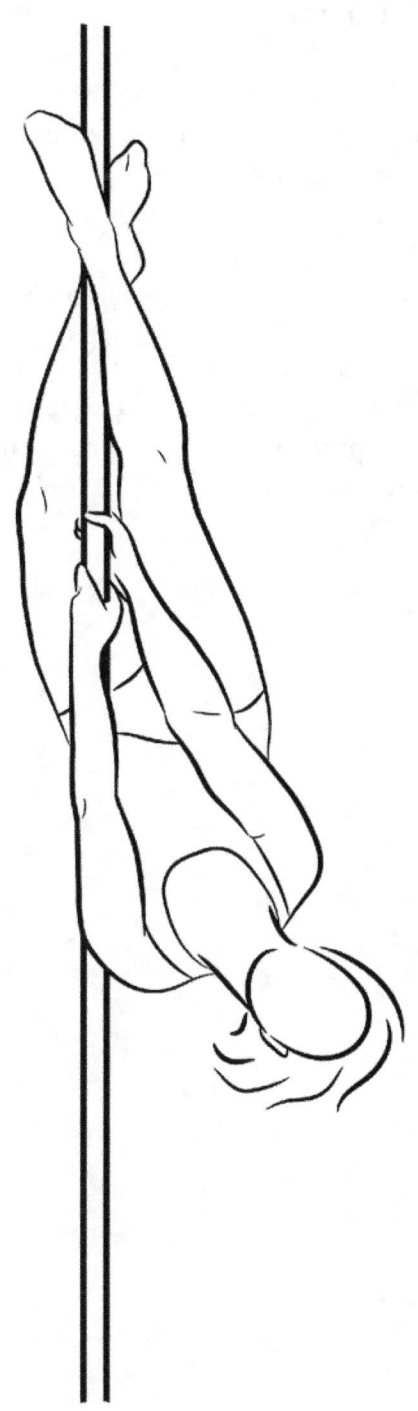

Cross Knee Release

This is a move that you can start from the ground. Instead of inverting, start off with a basic climb, getting as high as you can. From there, cross your legs together, creating a sitting position, having one thigh over the other. At this point, you can also create almost a right angle if you want to try that, but if not, slowly lean back and let go of the pole, using one hand at a time. Go all the way back, putting your arms out and arching your back.

Now, getting your hands off the pole is probably one of the scariest things you will attempt. We're often good at getting a leg or two out, but when it comes to letting your legs support you, it can be scary. It's imperative to go one leg at a time, so that you're not scaring yourself and doing this correctly in order to help overcome your fear.

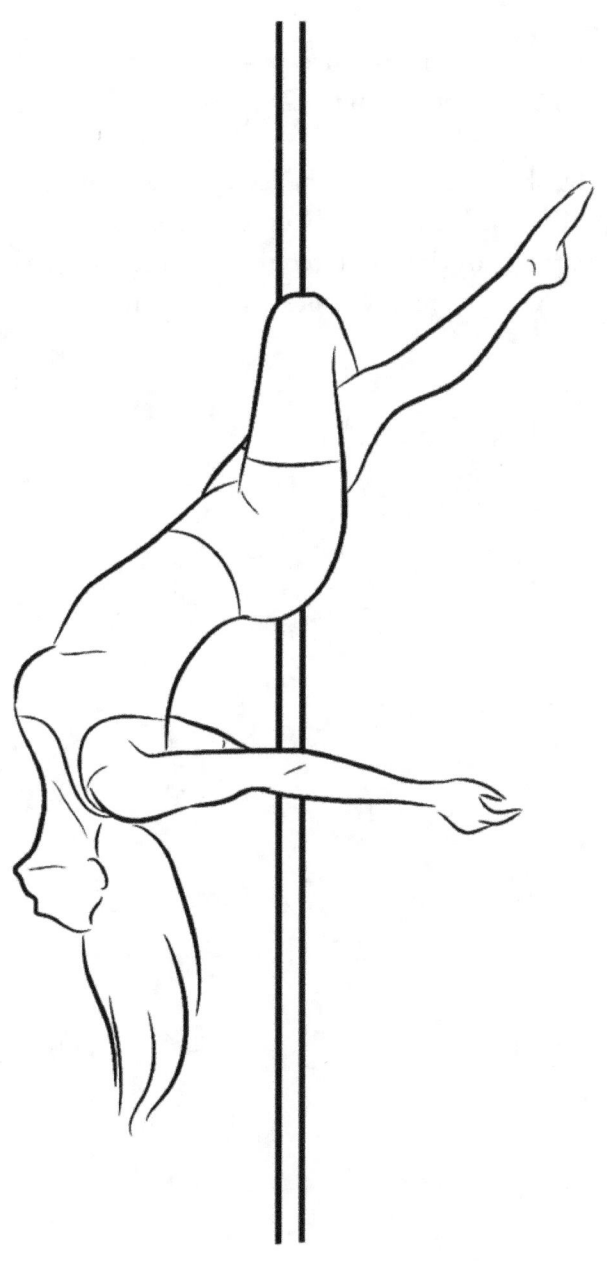

Sit-up Movement

Now, this is what you can do once you've inverted yourself. This can be complicated and does require a bit of leg and arm muscle strength. Now, the first step is to get inverted, and then take your leg off that is around the front of the pole. You should then take the leg that's around the back area of the pole. You should then lift your body up by using your arms to get into a leg cross or a pole sitting position. This requires extensive abs, so make sure you've been working on those ab muscles before you try this.

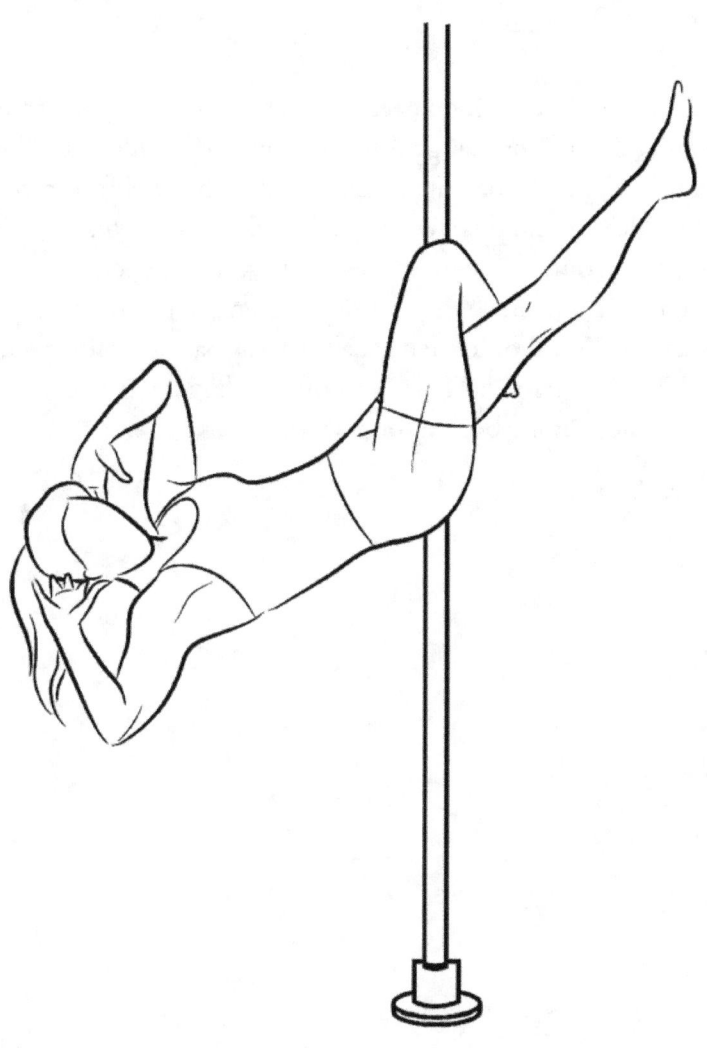

Cross Ankle

This is a variant of the crossing knees, but instead, you're going to be putting your ankles together in a crossing position. Your thighs will still be holding the brunt of your weight. To begin, you should do a basic climb to the top and then have your legs in the pike way, which is where you cross your ankles and have them straight out. You should then have your pole between your thighs, gripping it hard, and from there, you slowly lean your body back, taking one hand off at a time. You should then get all the way back, holding your arms out and keeping the back arched. This is a bit of a thigh killer initially, so make sure you work on conditioning before you try it.

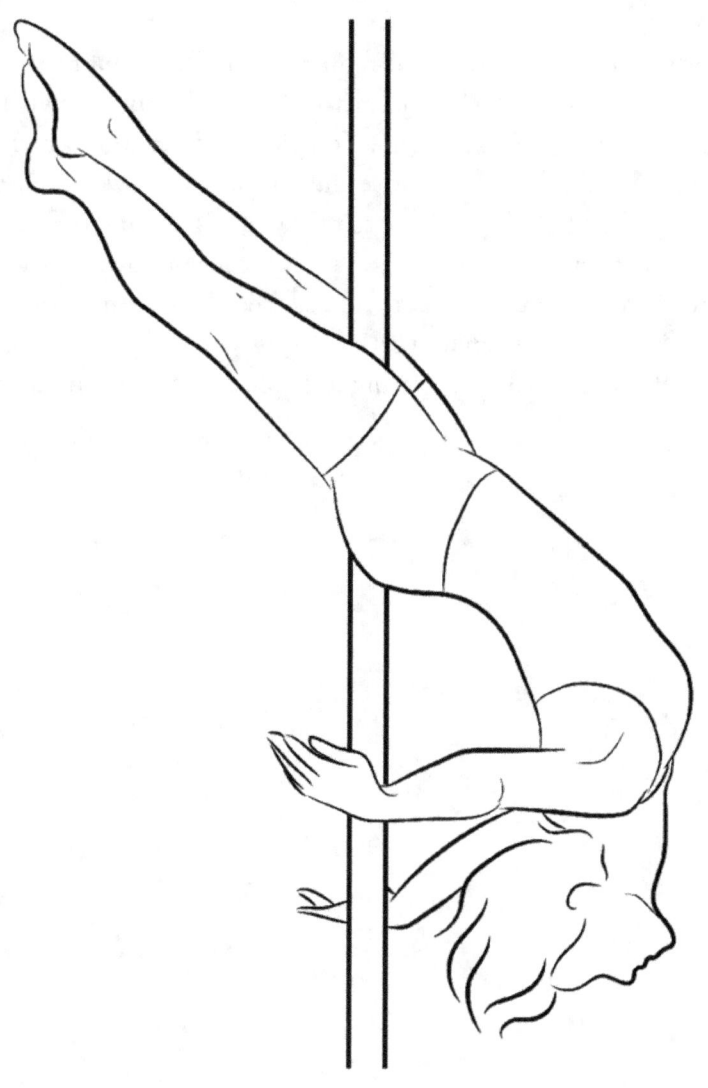

Butterfly

This is a fun little inverted move that requires you to have more arm and leg strength working together. To begin, start inverted, and then slowly take one of your hands and get it to a split grip. You should determine which leg will come off the pole beforehand and move the arm with it as well. For example, if you want your right leg off, you have to take your right hand off and move it slowly down. You should keep your hand with the leg on the pole there. Once you've changed this, point your toes and release the leg completely. Keep it bent and hold it there. This can be a bit daunting, especially if you don't move your hand down first, so work on getting to a split grip before you do this. It'll make it easier.

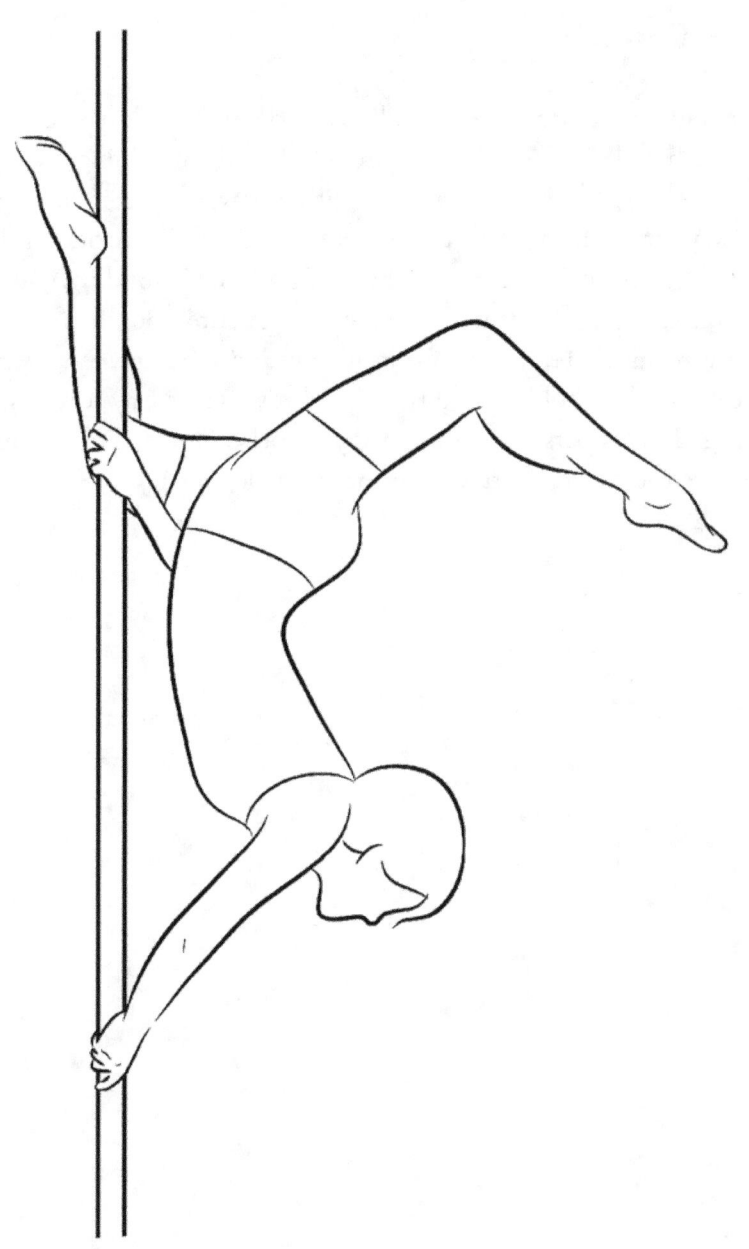

Inverted Crucifix

There are a few ways to do this. If you like to do handstands, you can do this from a reverse handstand position. For myself, I really like doing the inverted crucifix from a basic invert. You can start either way, but make sure you grip the pole with your thighs, holding them there. You should have one leg in front of the other leg, with one in front of the pole and one behind it. You should work to then cross at them at the ankles Make sure your legs are tightly squeezed, and from there, move your arms out and hold them at your sides. You can feel your legs holding you there, and it's a great way to work on leg conditioning. This is personally one of my favorite moves, and it's one that doesn't require too much effort, except for strong legs.

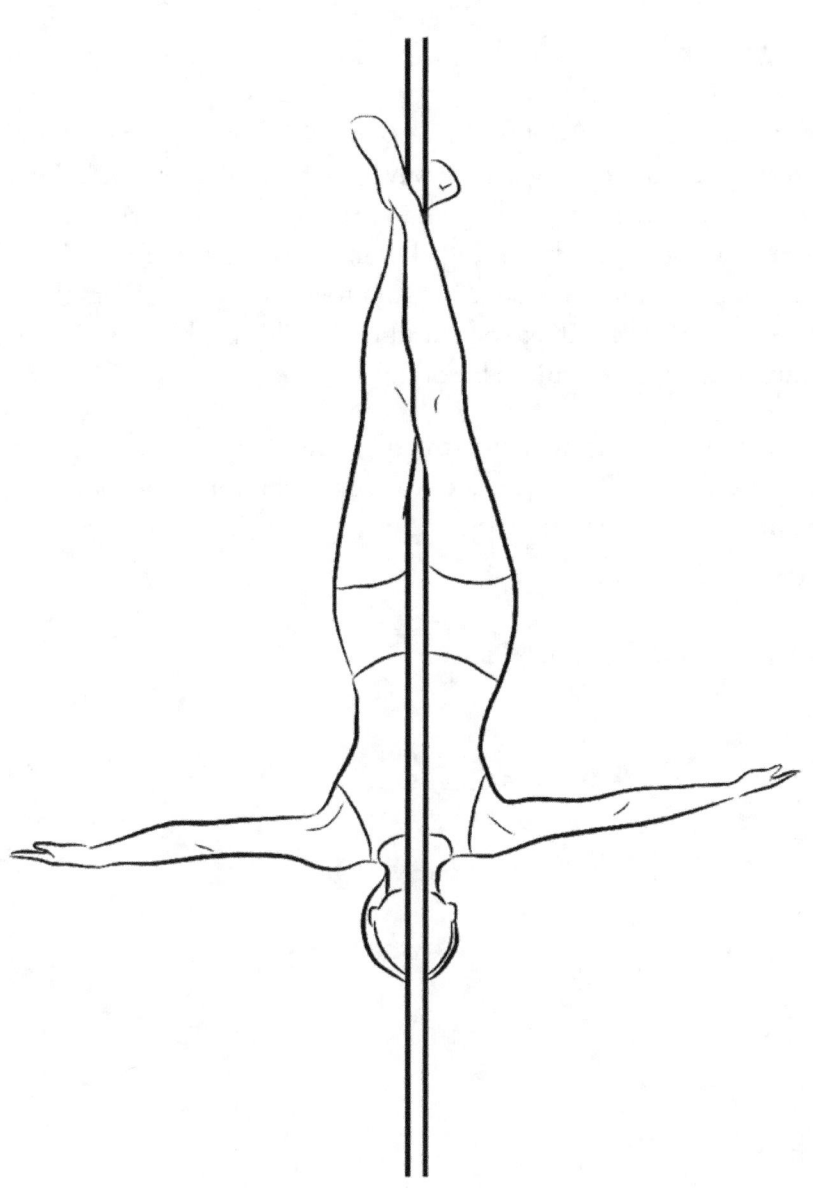

Brass Money

This is a variation in a sense of the inverted crucifix. You should start inverted, but instead of having your legs all the way straight, you should have them bent at the knee. You can climb up the pole in order to help make this look better, and from there, hold your hands together in a baseball grip. From there, keep your legs next to one another, pointing your toes, and holding them there. You should arch your back and let your head hang. This is a bit complicated, but once you get it down, it's quite a bit of fun.

These inversions are definitely worth trying out, and they can help up your pole game immensely. Try them, and work on them from time to time to help master these. Combine them with beginner moves for even more of a killer routine.

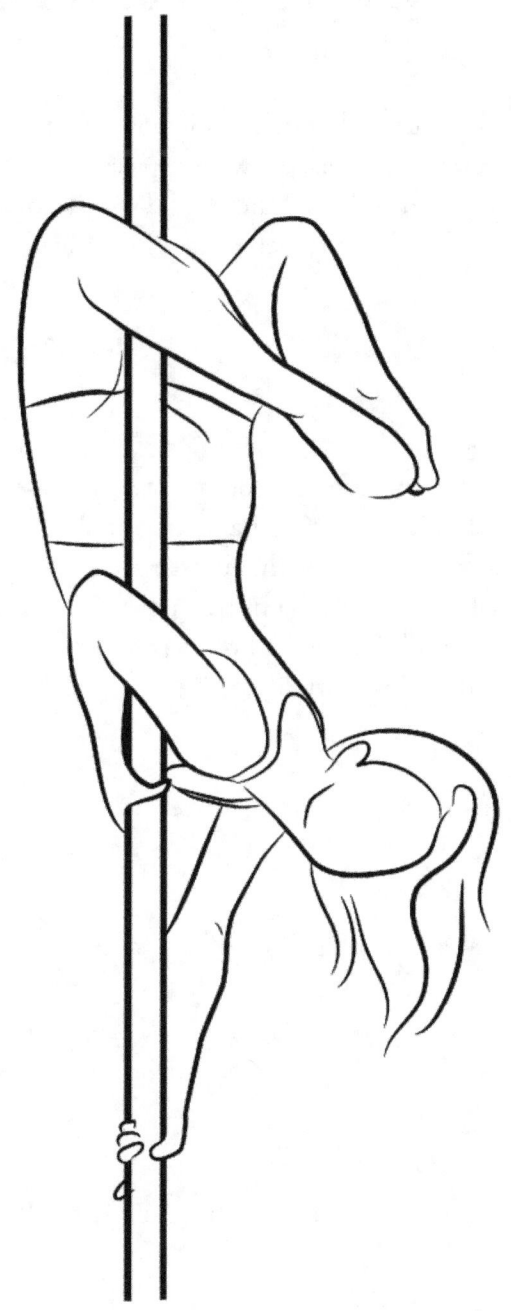

Intermediate Poses to Hold on a Pole

Now, some of you might be more interested in holding poses on a static pole. If you've been working mostly static, there are a few great poses to try out. This chapter will go over how to do each of these, and the best ways to do them. They're also good to help with intermediate inverts and other movements, too.

Handstand

This is your most basic pose to try, but often, if you're not a gymnast, this can be difficult. To do this, you should have your hands about shoulder width apart. Kick up your legs, and from there, let them rest against the pole. (Be careful so you don't accidentally slam them against the pole.) From there, you can grip it the pole, to help you hold the pose. This is a good post to work on if you're great at handstands but are bad with inverts.

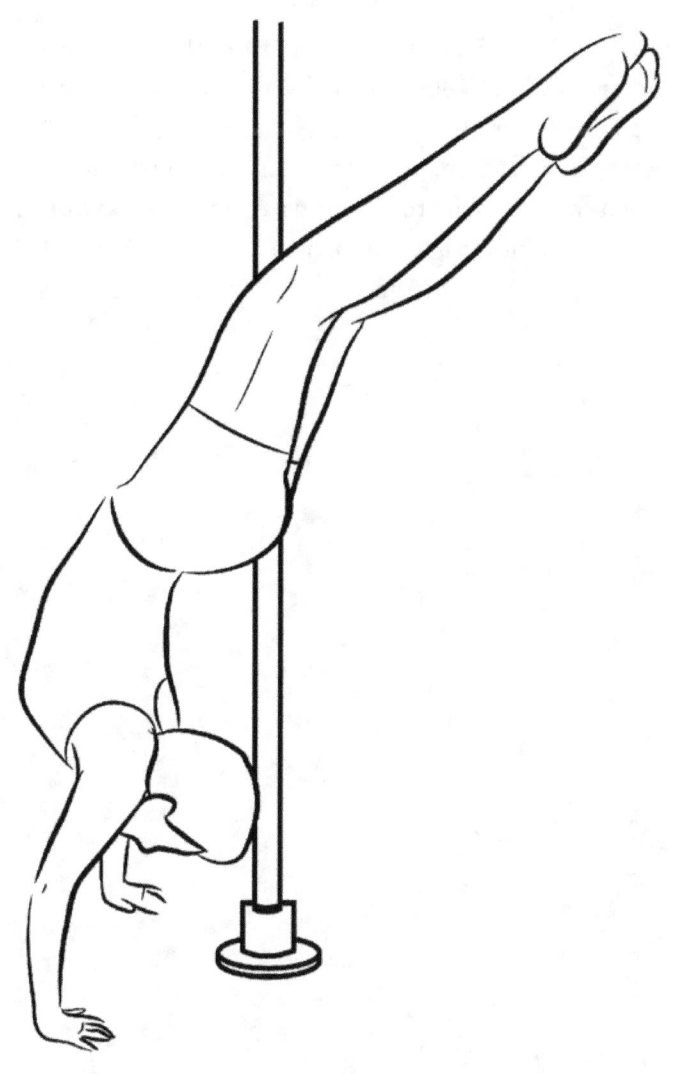

Reverse Handstand

You should be right against the pole, and from there you should then put your legs up and against the pole. You will want to use your feet to grip the pole, holding the stance. Your hands should be about the shoulder width apart. This pose is quite hard and often, it results in an occasional injury. You should make sure that if you're still trying to learn this, that you can start by having your legs against the pole and holding it, and from there, climb up with your hands until you're in the handstand position.

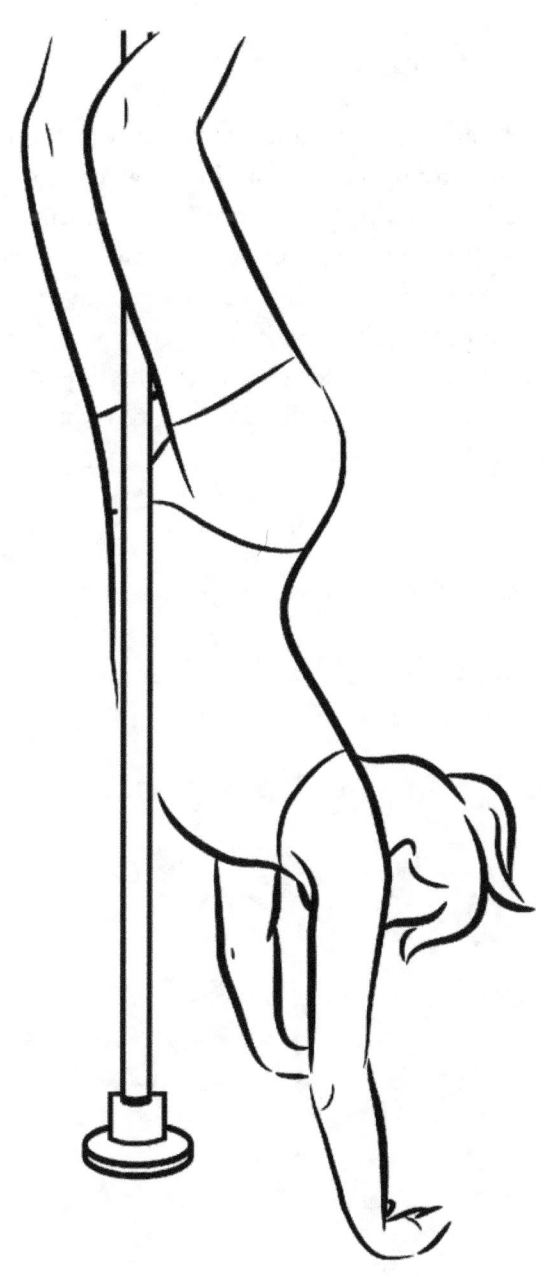

Bow and Arrow

This is another handstand variant. If you're wanting to work on holding yourself in a handstand position, or an invert where you only have one leg on the pole, then this is for you. To start, go into a normal handstand position, and from there, wrap your legs around the pole. From there, slowly take off your weaker leg of the two, and have your dominant leg wrap around the pole against your ankle, holding it there. From there, you can maintain this, keeping your posture secure, and your body straight. This does take a bit to get used to, but it's often a great exercise for those willing to try it.

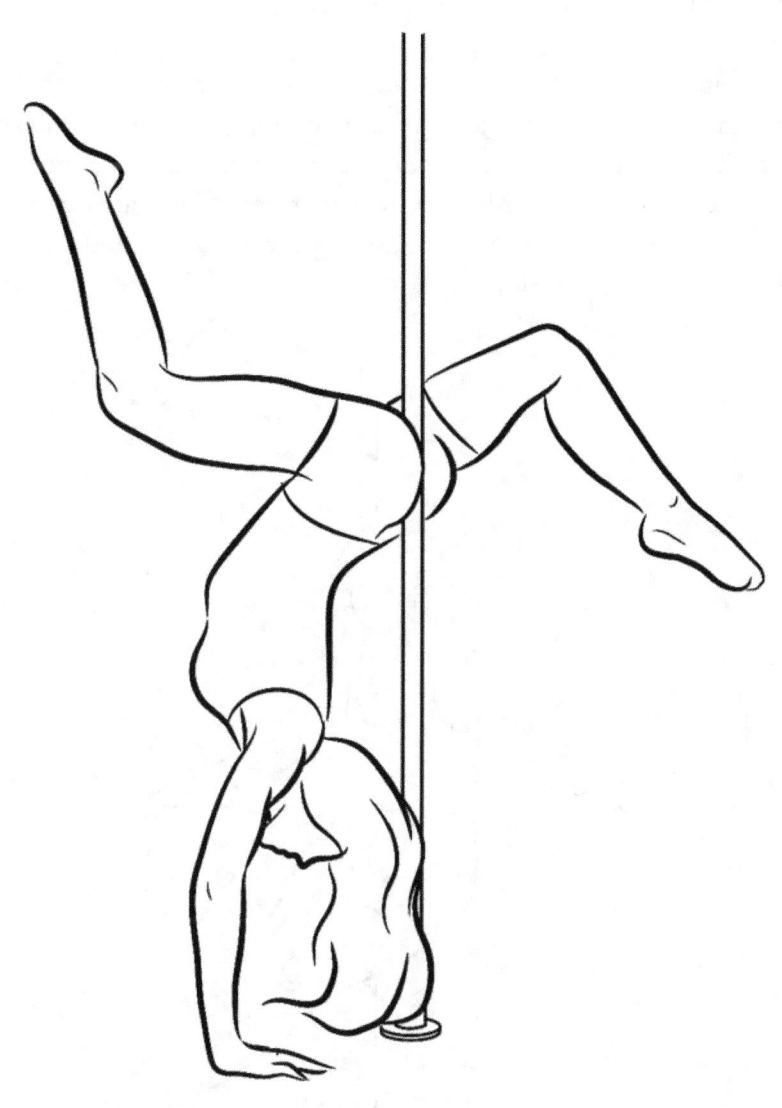

Peter Pan

This is a fun little pose to learn and for some, adding this to a combination in a routine makes it look amazing. To start, you simply get into a climb and hold your legs there. You should then wrap one leg in front of the pole and move it right next to the other one. Move your body forward so that your upper half of your body is in front of the pole. Extend your hands out and hold it there. To get out of this, just move your back to where it was before and slide down.

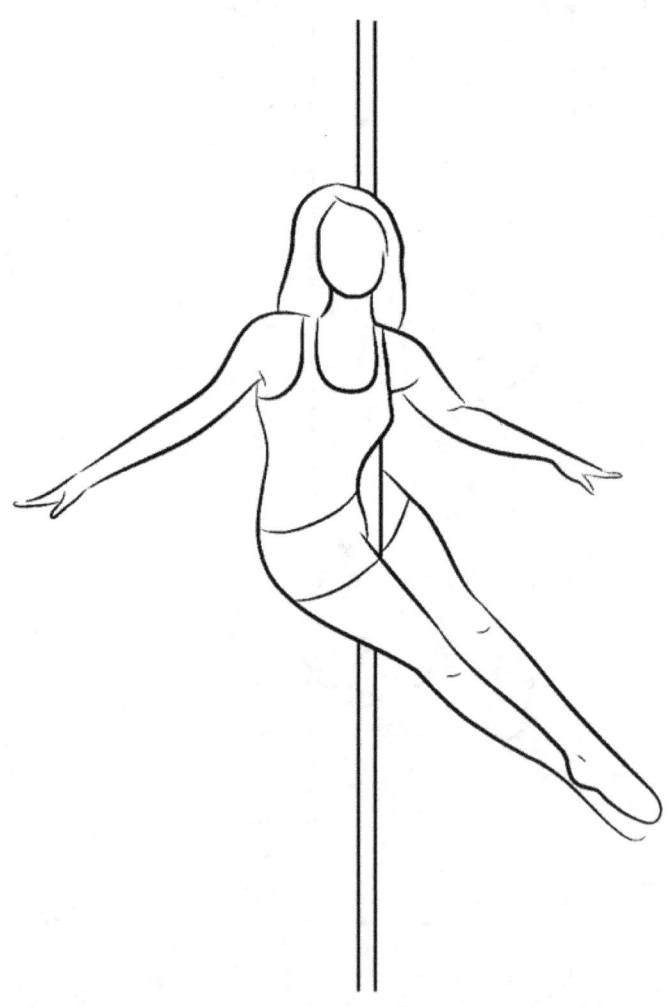

Jasmine

This is probably one of the hardest poses to learn. To start, you want to be in an inverted position. From there, you should then slide your body around to the side of your outer leg and hold it there. You should bend your knees; gripping the pole with your knee area together, and your hand holding it. You should then let your legs sit there.

If you want to do this with a straight leg (which is much harder), you should start from a normal invert. From there, wrap one leg around the pole and the other behind it. You should then let one of your arms fall down to the lower third of the pole and hold it there. Push your body out, and then let your hand hold it there. This pose is much harder than the bent leg, so master the bent leg before you move onto the jasmine.

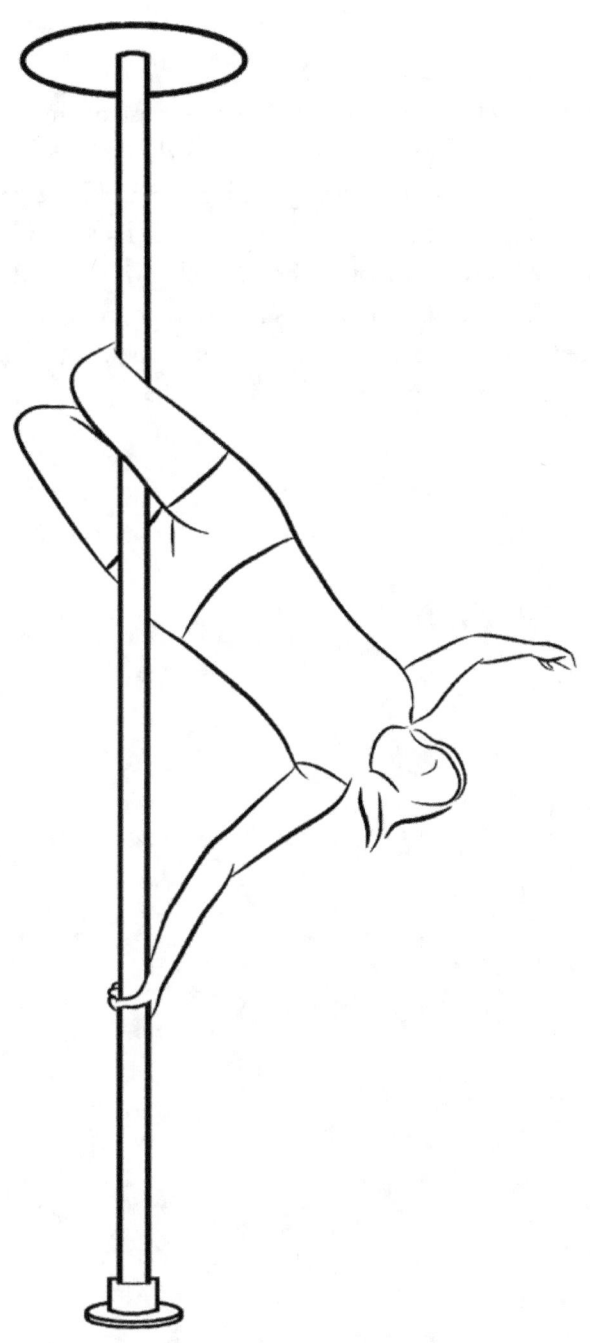

Layback

These are typically harder for people, not because of their nature, but because you must condition your body to let go off the pole. For this pose, start in a normal pike sit. You should bring your legs up and have your butt and legs at about the same level. For starting out, you can have your inner hand against the pole. Slowly move your other hand back, gripping the pole from behind. This can also be done with no hands if your legs are strong enough to grip the pole. Be forewarned though — that this can cause a lot of pain on your legs — if they're not conditioned.

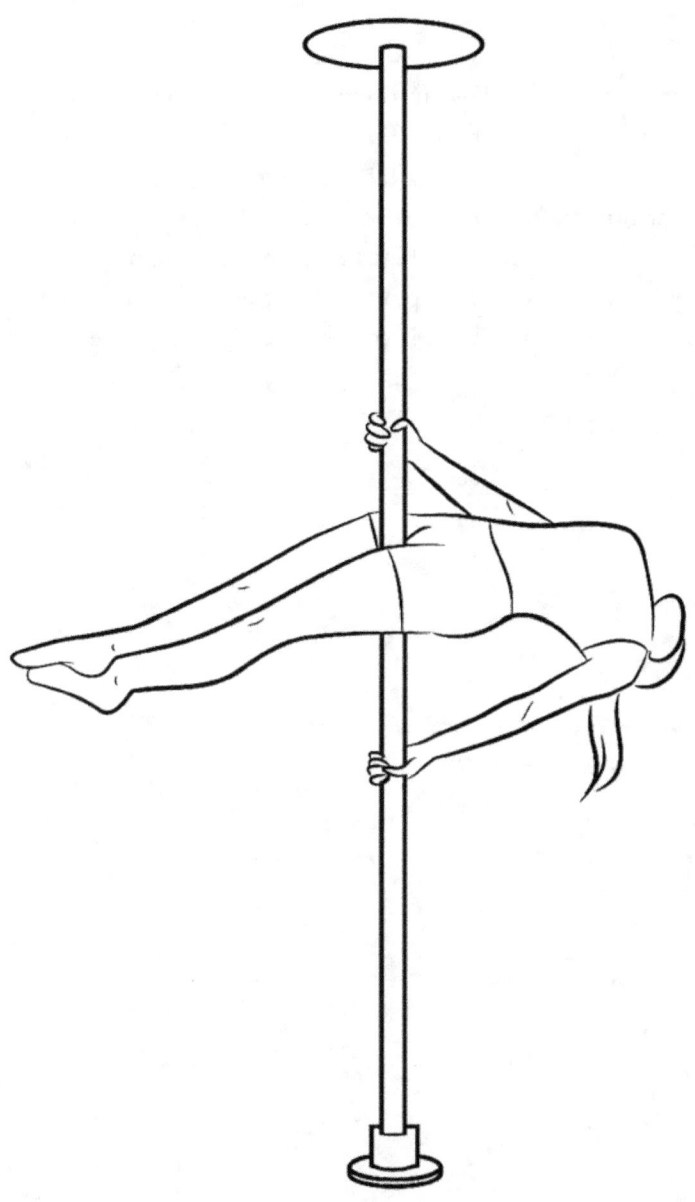

Armpit Hold

Did you know you can hold your body up with your armpits? Yes, you certainly can! You do this at first by having your right leg go up in a bent position against the pole, letting your left leg be straight against it. You should then have your armpit there, holding your body tightly. It's important to make sure that you're not too sweaty, since it can affect the grip on the pole. Hold it, and if needed, you can move your upper arm there as well to hold the pole more securely. This is a great sort of look if you want to have a nice added touch to a routine.

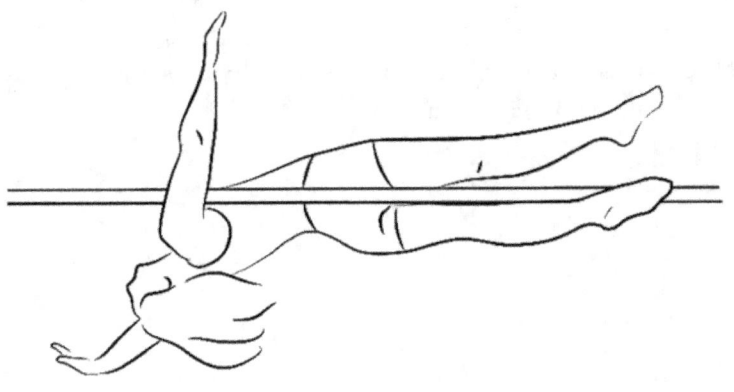

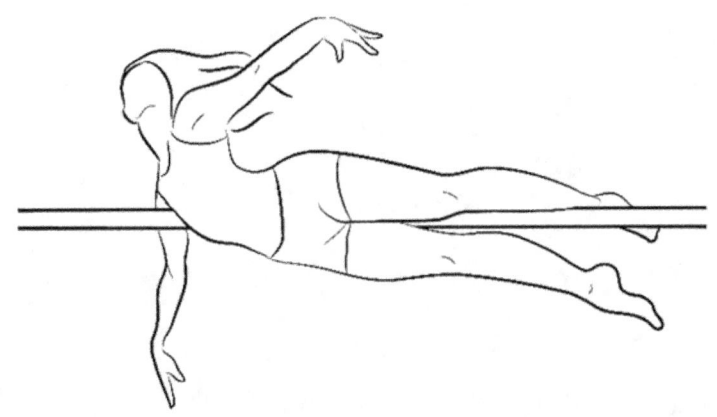

Elbow Grip

This is a hold that you can use either while spinning or not. To start, you should be in a normal pole position. From there, wrap your dominant hand against the pole, letting your elbow almost cradle against the pole. You can put your weight there, holding it to help build up strength. This is a great way to condition areas as well, making it easier on you.

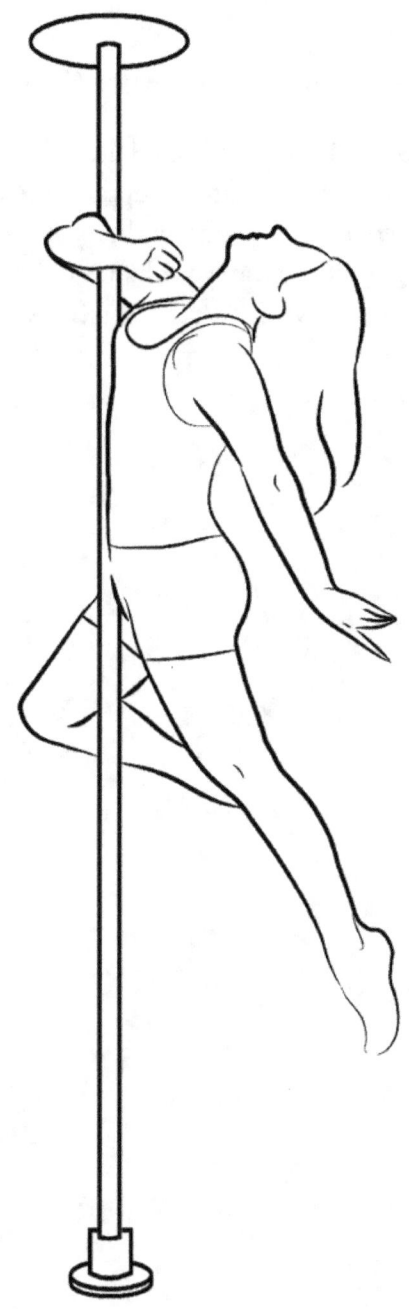

Bomb

This is a nice one if you want to have extra inverted action.

To start, get in the inverted position, and from there, pull your legs in. You can move the lower part of your legs forward, wrapping them around the pole. Typically, your thighs are what are holding you there, but you can also use your hands to grip the area. From there, wrap your hands either against the pole or around your body. You should work to get yourself as tightly tucked in as possible.

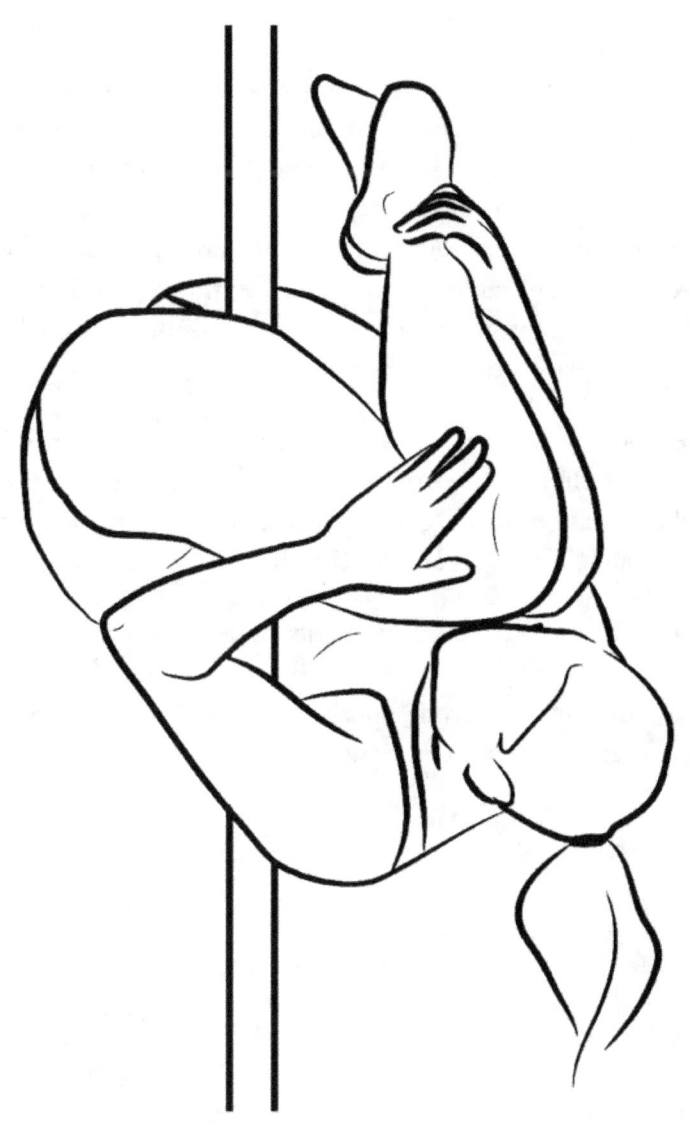

Cupid

Finally, there is the cupid. This one is super easy compared to the other two, but it's certainly something that you should try out. To begin, place your hand that is nearest to the pole up near the top, and then wrap that same leg around, holding your knee there to help support the area. From there, lean back, using the knee and arm to support your body weight, and bring your other leg up to help straighten yourself. Hold it, and you'll feel the grip and tension against your legs. This is great for some back-of-the-knee conditioning, which is often one of the hardest places to strengthen.

Most of these poses are great to try out to help you with conditioning of your body, and also to help you once you start to do more advanced moves. You can use these when you're practicing, and often, they can assist you if you struggle with grips and such. Try them and see the difference they make.

It's encouraged to try these poses in static mode at first. That way, you can work on holding your body weight up while staying static. For many, this is a great way to also improve your spins, for these can be used with other techniques to create gorgeous combos.

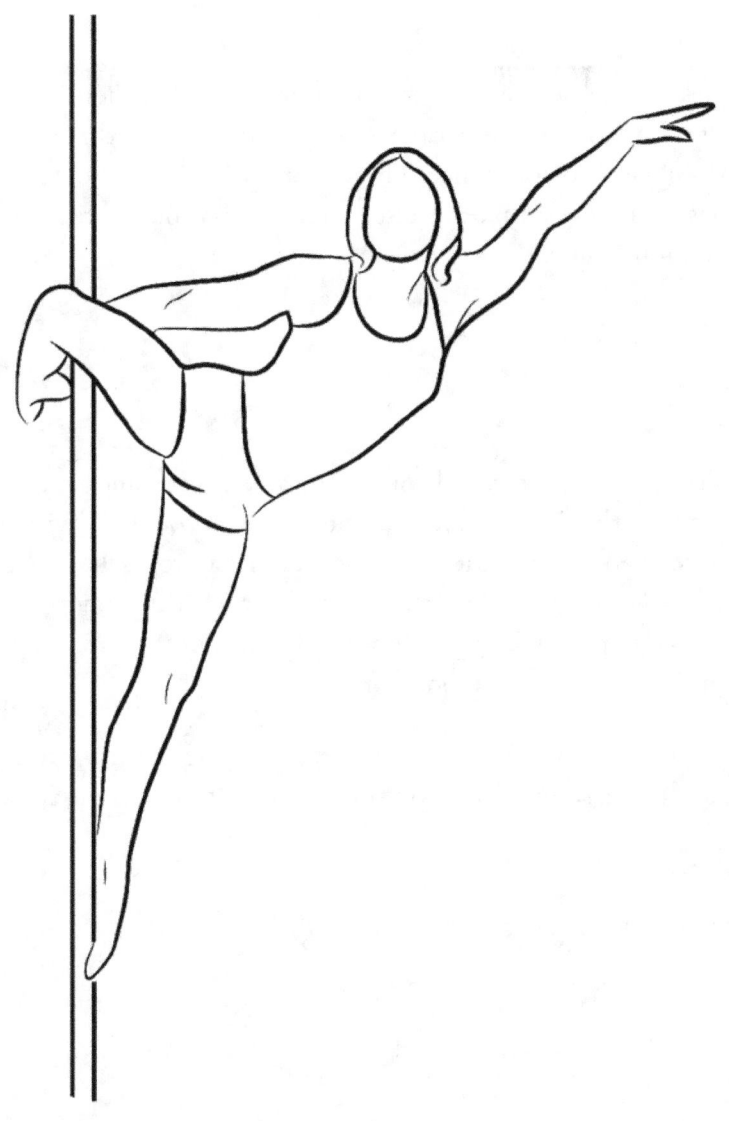

Intermediate Slides and Floor Work

While poses can be done while holding onto the pole, there are still some amazing slides and other floor work to help you do the best that you can when you're learning how to pole dance. This chapter will tell you how to do each of these moves, and these simple exercises can also help you create a great combo that will certainly shine.

Dive Up

This is one that looks pretty, and you will be able to get some great abdominal engagement with this. To start, you should be flat on your back with your arms held out, stretched to each side of the floor, holding yourself up. You should then start to slowly move your back in an arching position and from there, use the abdominals to push your upper body from the floor. You should continue to hold your back in an arched position.

If you really want to try something complex, try doing this from your pole and hold yourself there, sliding your body down to create a gorgeous look.

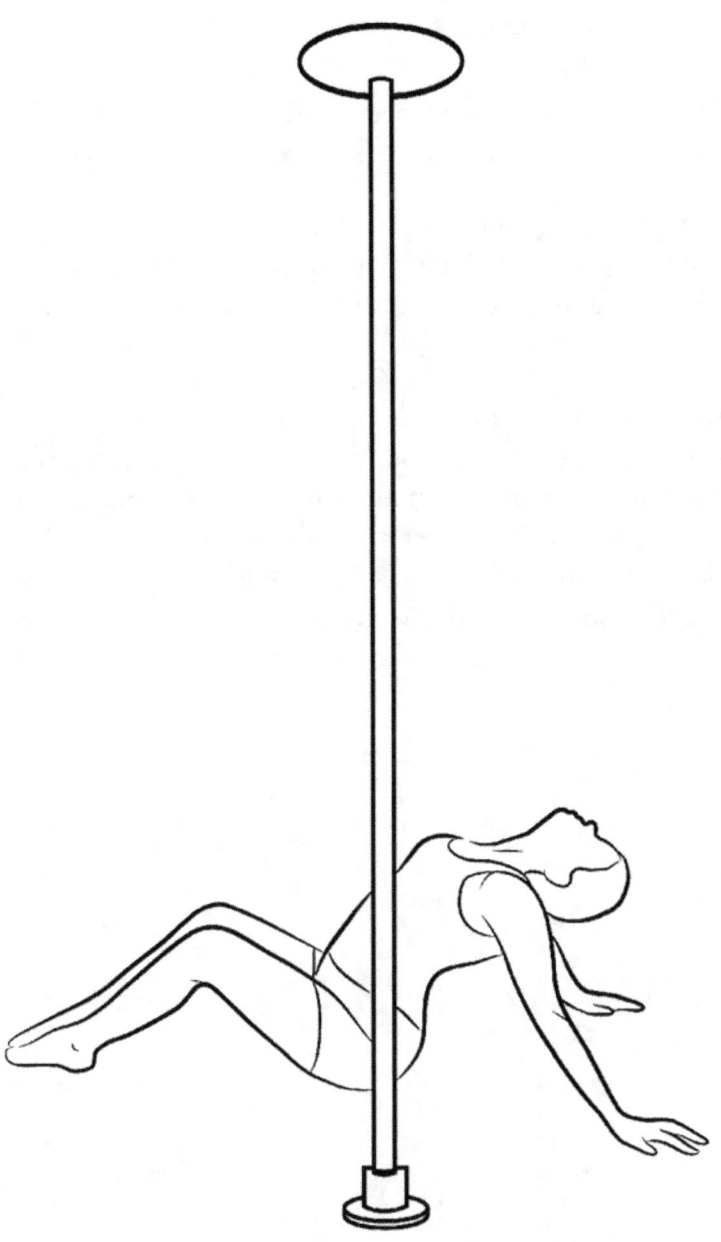

Prance Shoulder Mount

The shoulder mount was discussed in an earlier chapter, but if you're looking for a pretty piece of floor work, now is the time.

You're not actually going to be doing a shoulder mount with this one, but instead, you'll be holding your body there in the grip, beginning to kick your leg straight up, trying to get as close to the ceiling as possible. That's the goal you want to achieve.

However, instead of using just one leg, have your second leg move straight behind you, doing it closely behind the other one. You can do these kicks again and again, and often, if you're struggling with the shoulder mount, you should try doing these first to help you get a feel for using your shoulders in that fashion. It does help a lot, and it can make a difference in how you move. It's a nice piece of added floor work, too, in order to help you look even better.

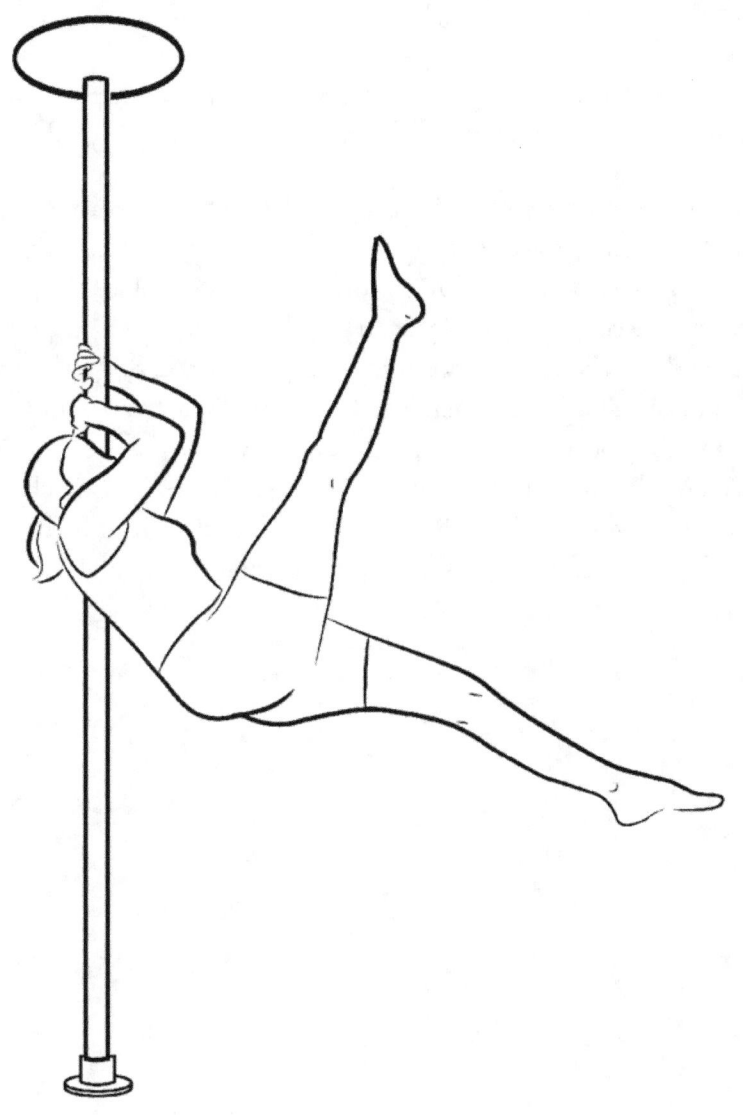

Wrist Seat

This is a slide that requires you to have a lot of arm strength, so if you don't have that yet, work on the other movements before you try this.

To begin, you should start by climbing the pole as high as you can comfortably go. You should strive to go to the top, but if you're not able to due to the nature of what you have to do next, that's totally understandable. When you get to the place you're comfortable with, you should then let go of the pole with your weaker hand and then have it positioned slightly further down the pole, almost like a split grip. You should then lean back a bit and extend your legs. Make it into a straddling position as you slowly slide down the pole. It's also imperative that you do point your toes, to make this look prettier and much more fluid. If you are struggling with anxiety about holding this from higher up on the pole, it's best that you start from a lower position. It will make it much easier on you.

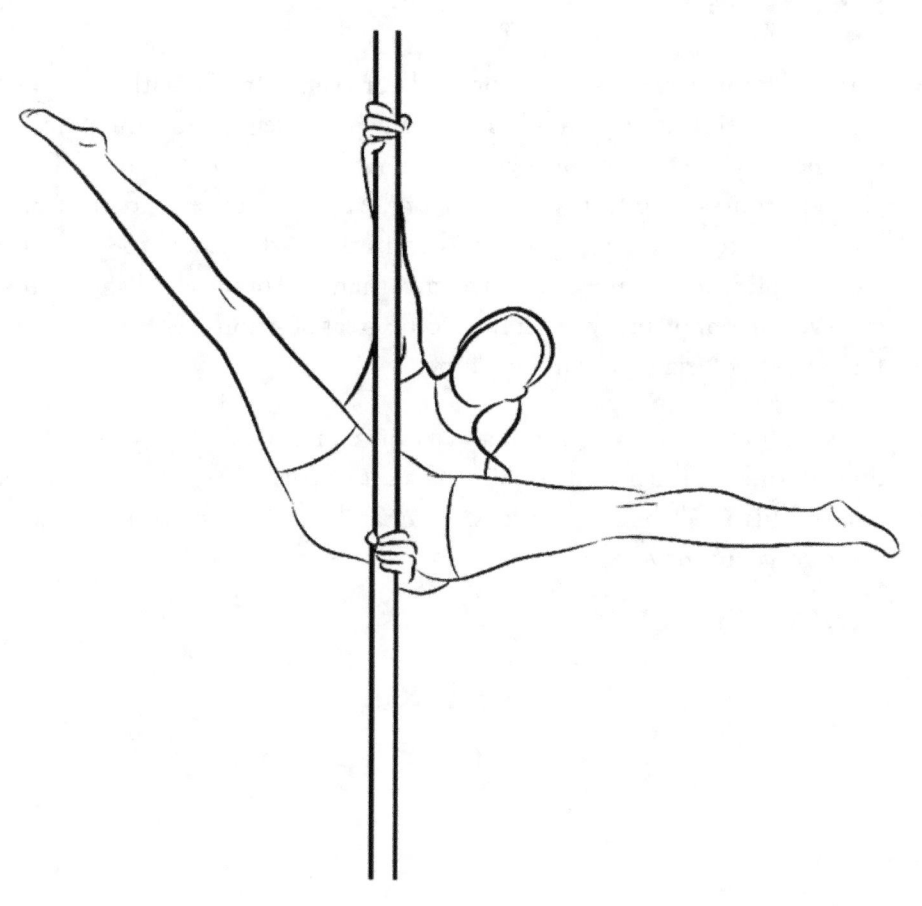

Side Climb

This can be an extra piece of floor work, or even help you with your position. To begin with this, you should have your inside leg around the pole, having your hands close to one another in a strong-hold grip. Pull your body up and have your outside leg against the back of the pole. You're essentially using your knee inside to start, leading up, and from there, the straight leg will follow. This requires much more arm strength than the other climbs, but this also gives you an opportunity to get into some great positions, which will definitely make your pole dancing combos shine.

These various extras are great to add to any combination that you'd like. They do take time to learn, and you'll need a bit of patience. But once you get the hang of this, you'll be able to use these in tandem with everything else to create some gorgeous movements.

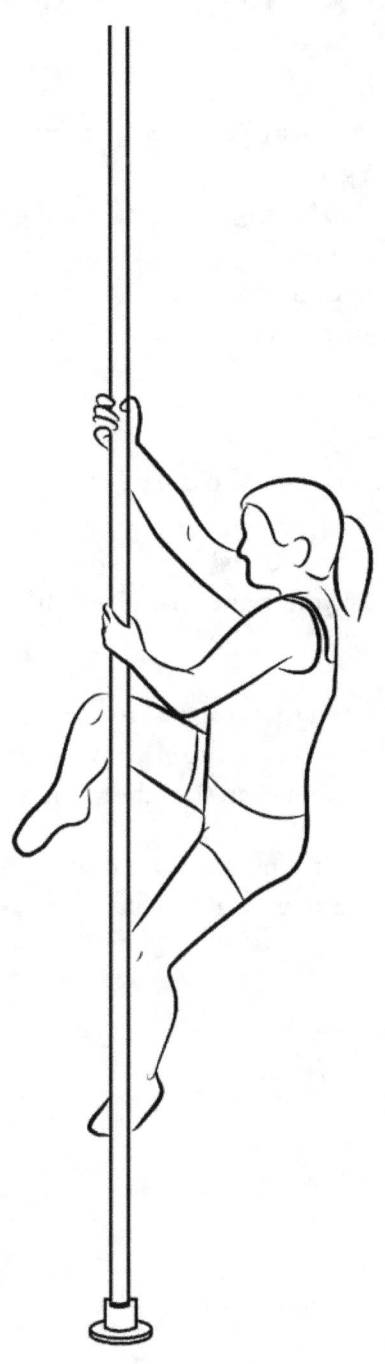

The Shoulder Mount

One of the other moves that many people want to try is the shoulder mount. Now shoulder mounts are good, but they do carry with them a bit of danger, mostly because people tend to fall when they start doing these. But, if you want to get better, you should certainly try to make sure you do these. There are a few safety tips that we'll go over, along with how to do these. They will help you improve and become successful.

How to Do a Shoulder Mount

To begin, we'll go over how you do this. When you start, you should have your back touching the pole, with your spine on one side. It's best to keep it on your dominant side.

You should then take the hand that is closest to the pole into a cup grip that is above where your inner shoulder is. A cup grip is with your fingers and thumbs on the same side with the thumb nearest to the ground.

Next, take the outer arm — the one that's not nearest to the pole — and have that in a cup grip right above your head height.

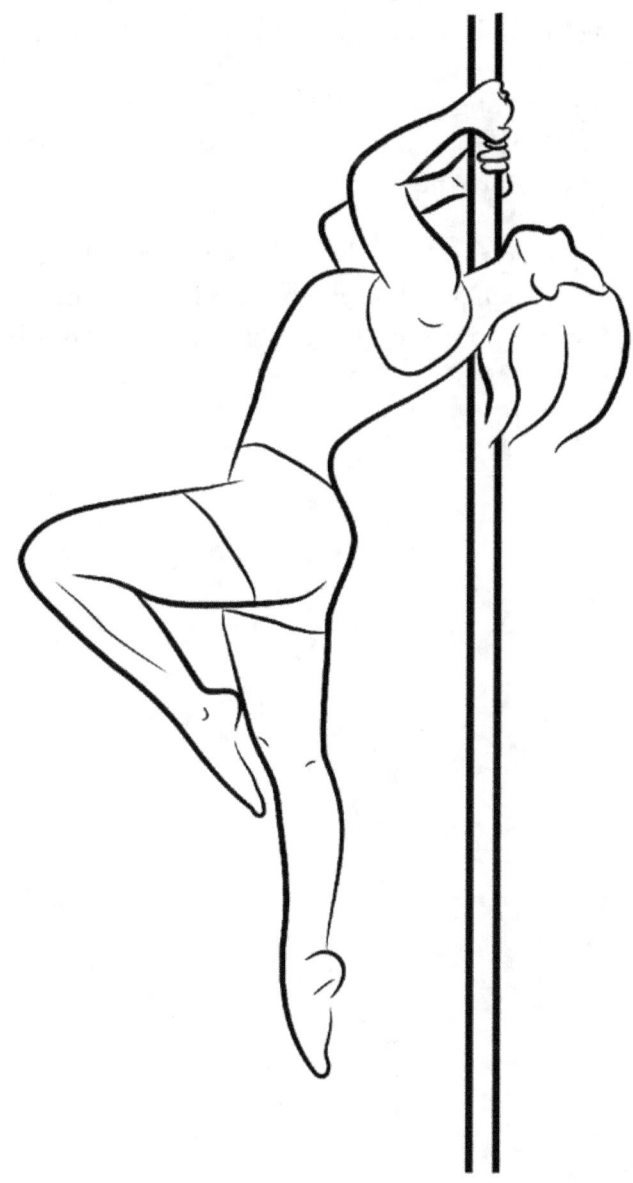

You should then pull the pole. The best way to do this is to visualize what you're doing. Imagine that you're going to throw your pole across the room. Obviously, you won't, but when you do this, you will have your elbows start to come near one another as you begin to pull. You need to maintain contact between the pole and your shoulder at all times. You should look up.

When you are first learning, you should have your inner foot in front and your outside behind where the pole is, which is on the outside of the pole. This will help you with moving into the next position.

From there, you should then take the back leg that is against the pole up and move it towards the ceiling and where the pole is. move your legs so that the outside leg is in front, and the inside leg is behind you. This will take you to a basic invert grip.

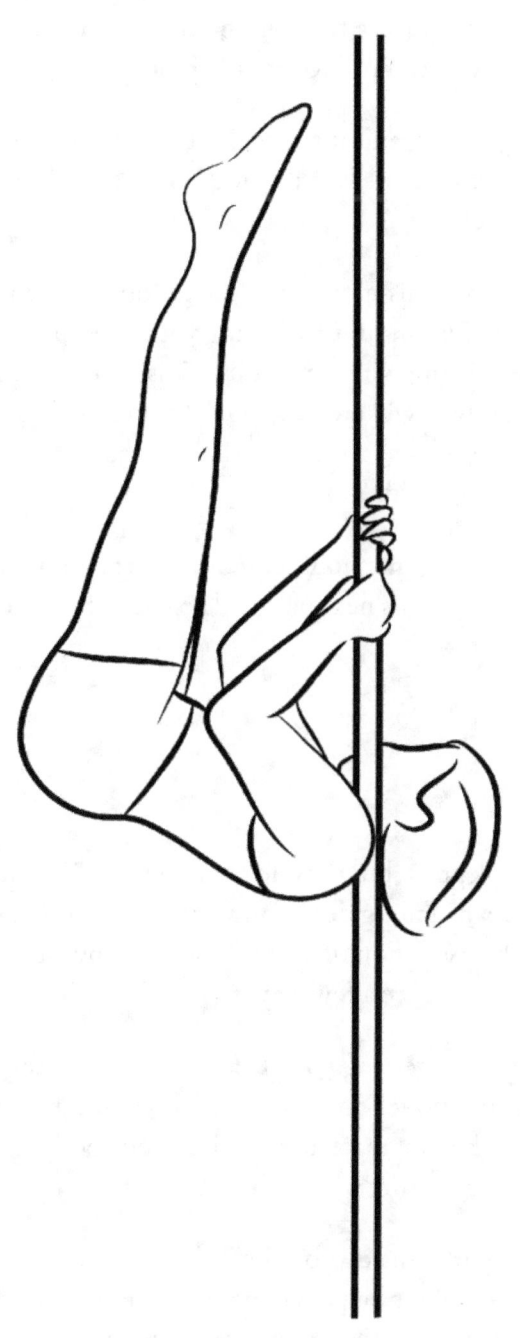

You should from there, squeeze the legs and have your collarbone move away from the pole so that you can roll to face the pole.

This takes a lot of practice, and it's very hard to get used to. This is probably the hardest move in this entire book. But if you master this, it will definitely boost your confidence!

Now, if you've mastered this move with the leg outside behind the pole, you can do a deadlift shoulder mount by having your feet apart in front of where the pole is and then lifting with your hips. This takes a lot more abdominal strength, but ultimately, it will create a much crisper look to your movements. If making sure that you have a fluid motion is what you're looking for, you should definitely consider this move.

Now that you know about the shoulder mount, there are a few things that you should keep in mind, and this next part will go over a few safety tips for you to learn.

Safety Tips

Shoulder mounts look great, but they do come with their own fair share of risk. The biggest risk is really falling down on your head or on your shoulder. The worst many get is a bruised shoulder, and I've gotten my fair share of pole kisses from this. However, there are a few ways to help with this.

If you're struggling with getting your feet up, try doing the shoulder mount prances. These are mentioned in a future chapter, and they're a great way to help you get used to kicking back and leading your body up. You should try these if you're really struggling with shoulder mounts.

If you're worried about falling on your head, look at the environment of where your pole. Is. It's best to not be pole dancing on hardwood floors period, but it's even more imperative when you're trying to master a shoulder mount. Ideally, if you need to do it on a hardwood surface, you should make sure that you have mats set around the area, so that you don't end up bonking your head or your shoulders, causing pain.

It's best not to focus an entire pole session on the shoulder mount. Yes, you really want to learn it, but it takes a lot of practice and technique, and for some, you might end up working on this all the time and not getting anywhere. That's why it's imperative to not focus your entire practice on this. Yes, a bit of time dedicated to shoulder mounts is a great thing, but it's also good to make sure that you do focus on other inverts and spins as well, just so that you don't feel yourself getting discouraged.

Shoulder mounts are hard and they're not something you can just pick up in a day. Unless you've got killer abdominals and you do pull ups with inverts at the gym constantly, you won't be able to master these right off the bat. It requires a complex grip. It's best to make sure that if you're feeling frustrated, to stop, work on something else, and from there come back to this. Shoulder mounts will still be there when you get back, and you should learn them when you're at your strongest.

It's also important to learn your grips. The cup grip is what you use with the shoulder mount and it's important that you don't try to do any other grips. That's because the invert was made to hold your body up like that. If you're doing it otherwise, you could end up hurting your wrist because you're twisting it in a way you're not used to, which could potentially leave you open for injuries. Do make sure that you don't try to do any other grips with this but a cup grip.

Now, shoulder mounts can be a bit scary to try, and often, they are something most pole dancing enthusiasts want to learn. If you're going to take these on, do remember the safety tips and how to apply them. Make sure that you're doing some abdominal exercises as well, for that is where of your movements will be focused. By learning how to do these moves properly and taking your time to effectively learn how to move your body in this fashion, you'll be able to feel the effects, including the difference in the way your body feels with every single motion. It's a very pretty move, one that does look elegant, but just remember that in order to look that elegant, you need to practice.

Intermediate Does Not Mean Easy

You've learned in this book some intermediate pole dancing actions. Now, this is often where many people get stuck when they're learning, because even these intermediate motions do take a bit of time to get used to and they're often very hard.

However, you don't have to settle for this. You can get better and with every single move, if you practice it again and again, you'll feel the results. Often, it does require other physical strength as well, so if you weren't doing abdominal work or arm work, then it might be best to consider doing it. However, you can also achieve this from learning the movements alone, which is pretty nifty.

With this book, you've learned many key pole dancing grips and movements. This is the foundation for many of the harder pole dancing moves and it's often something that many people aspire to work on. So, if you begin this, your next step is to practice these moves again and again. You might end up having to practice these a hundred times before you truly get the hang of it. Even so, once you do get a feel for this, and once you learn it, you'll immediately see and feel the difference. This book is the next place you turn to if you've mastered beginner moves. Hopefully, as you continue on your pole dancing journey, you'll master these moves as well.

Win a free

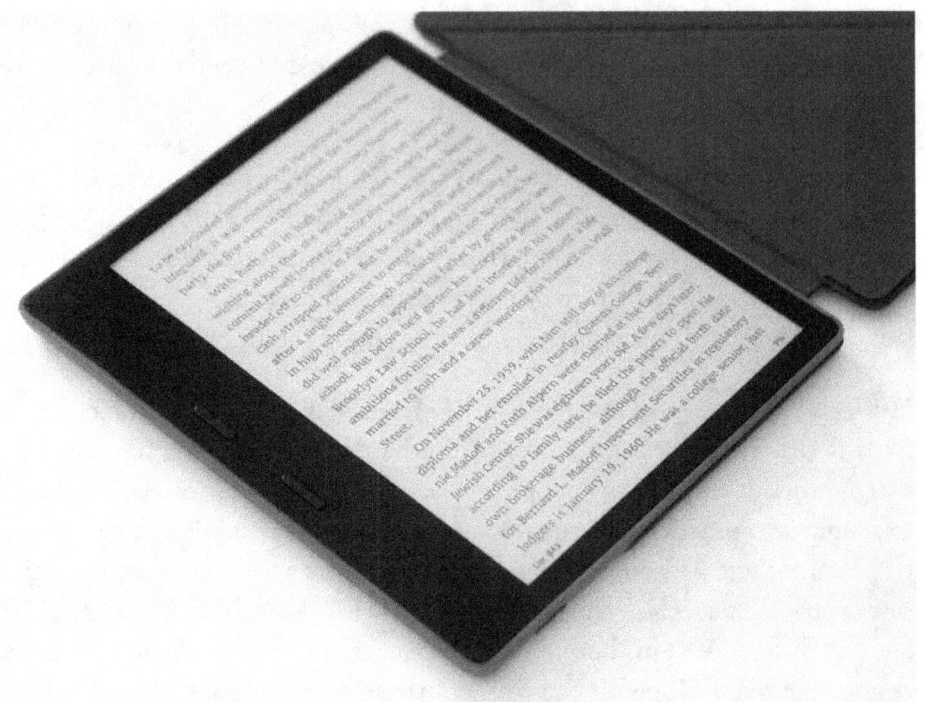

kindle
OASIS

Let us know what you thought of this book to enter the sweepstake at:

http://booksfor.review/intermediatepole

Want to take your pole dancing to the **next level**?

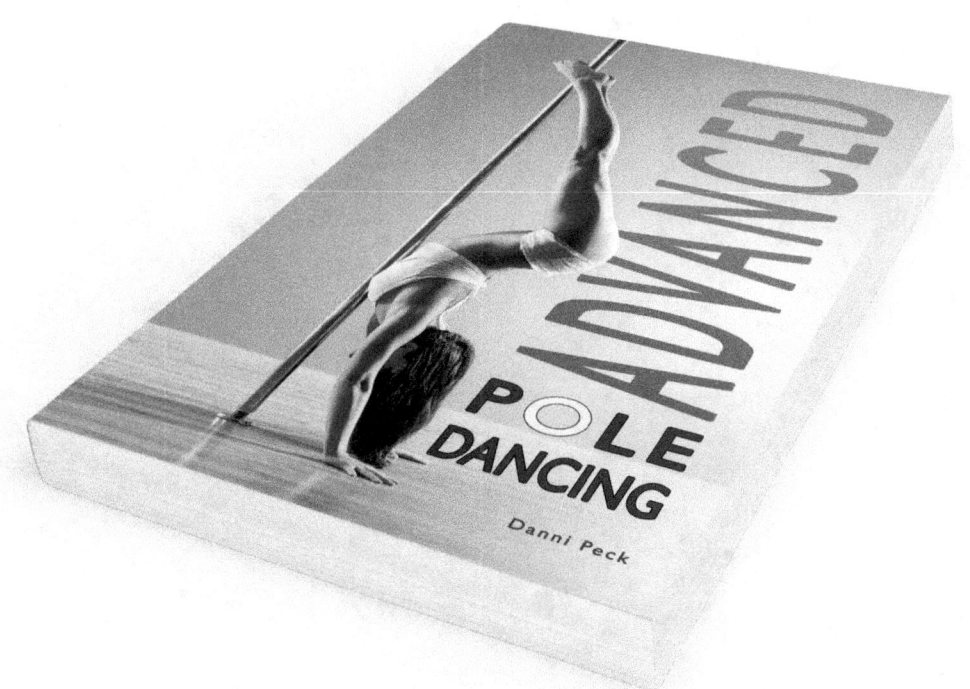

Advanced Pole Dancing
For Fitness and Fun

Available on Amazon

Page intentionally left blank